D1562997

BLACK MEN IN DENIAL?

CHALLENGING SOCIAL BELIEFS ON BLACK MEN AND PROSTATE CANCER

*The Benefits of Increasing Awareness,
Early Diagnosis and Intervention*

Ali Abdoul

Public Health Community Inclusion Specialist

Disclaimer

This publication and its contents are provided for informational purposes only. All information and ideas are provided in good faith or opinion of the author, and the author's research findings. To the best of the author's knowledge and experience, the information is true and honest.

The author, reserve the right to vary or change any such opinions subsequently. It is impossible to provide comprehensive information and advice tailored to each situation within a publication such as this. Therefore, it should not be regarded as any kind of substitute for appropriate and personalised professional advice. Nothing in this publication can be used as a promise or guarantee. Adoption, implementation or trial of any of the information, ideas, methods or systems mentioned in this publication and on the associated website are the reader's choice. You, the reader, are totally responsible for the choices and decisions you make, and for all consequences of those decisions. I apologise for any errors, omissions or inaccuracies that may be found in this document.

I aim to produce easy to read, short books and other publications that will empower and encourage high-performance, personal and professional development for all people regardless of race, creed, colour, sexual orientation or religion. I hope you find it useful and empowering. Furthermore, I hope it helps towards reaching your highest level of achievement and handling all your goals with the purpose and dynamism of a 'sports person'!

Editing and Layout: Amina Chitembo & the Diverse Cultures squad.

Cover Designed: Ahsan Chuhadry, Graphics Designer

Main photo of Ali Abdoul: Amina Chitembo

Published by Diverse Cultures Publishing, UK.

Website: www.diverse-cultures.co.uk

Email address: publishing@diverse-cultures.co.uk

Postal Address: 28–29 Maxwell Road, Peterborough, PE2 7JE.

Paperback ISBN: 978-0-9957396-7-3

Dedication

To my wife Amina, my daughters Naila and Iman, my stepdaughters Ngosa and Ngweshe who, each in their own ways, remind me of the value of life. I appreciate the love, laughter and meaning they bring to mine. May God continue to bless every one of them.

SUBSCRIBE TO MY BLOG:

Get more training, tools and tips from me and other thought leaders on Inclusion issues:

https://www.aliabdoul.com

I will see you there.

—Ali.

Contents

Introduction

> *"It is not until we the co-conspirators stand up and share to help ourselves shall we start to see the beauty of living in a caring community."*
> *~Ali Abdoul.*

It is 2018, and still, many conversations are going on about black men's health inequalities or non-inclusion. I always hear questions such as:

Why are more black men dying pre-maturely of prostate cancer, testicular cancer and indeed any other cancers?

Why is it that so many black men are burying their heads in the sand, and not seeking help early enough to increase their chances of treatment when they develop Prostate Cancer?

Why are we not talking about it?

Is it another 'white man's' disease that doesn't affect us men of colour?

Some people maybe even believe that we are cursed, or that we are unlucky. The truth is, a lot is going on in the black man's mind. The beliefs, upbringing, and fear are just the starting point. Many of us black men are well educated and hold very good jobs, but still, we don't seem to want to seek help when it comes to our health and wellbeing.

Are we experiencing barriers to services?

Or are we just not brave enough to know the results and instead pass it off as a 'white man's' diseases?

The fact is that the odds are stacked against us. There are disparities in health outcomes for black men. Black men are more likely to die prematurely from prostate cancer than men from other communities. The statistics show that there is a one in four chances of black men having prostate cancer in their lifetime and dying from it against one in eight for the rest of the population.

Health inequalities have been an issue that governments after governments, policies after policies have been trying to grapple with. Reports have been written; strategic document produced, and programmes initiated. However, the effects have not been important enough.

They have been defined as the differences in health status between different population groups, mainly when those differences are unfair and avoidable. These inequalities do not occur by chance but are socially determined by circumstances largely beyond an individual's control. These circumstances disadvantage people and limit their chance to live longer healthier and fulfilling lives.

Health inequalities are said to be caused by the uneven distribution of income, power and wealth, which can lead to poverty and marginalisation of individuals and communities.

In this book, I explore the issue of prostate cancer in black men, the perceptions, the barriers, the interventions and I challenge some social beliefs.

As part of my master's degree in Public Health, I was looking for a topic to research. I wanted to write about something that would increase knowledge and awareness to me and the future generation in black and Minority Ethnic (BME) communities.

Before you start thinking I am a medical doctor, I will start by telling you about why I am so keen on this subject. I am tackling this issue from a community and social development point of view which is my specialism. As a black man, I am

challenging our beliefs, stereotypes, and norms that
we black men carry of being the last ones to seek
help when we have problems. As a Public Health
Inclusion specialist, I provide consultancy training
and speaking to help fellow practitioners find ways
of working with men from black and Minority
Ethnic communities

I chose to research Prostate Cancer, especially in black men because the issue has a particular meaning to me and the community. Not
only would I make an invaluable contribution to
addressing such big problem that is a taboo subject in many countries, but I would also contribute
to increasing a much-needed knowledge base for
myself and future generations.

Although I found the journey exciting and
the experience very illuminating, at first, I did not
have any idea about the extent of the problem of
prostate cancer in black men.

However, I set to research and learn more
about it. What I found was startling.

The aim of this book is:

1. To raise awareness, not only to black men
   but to their wives, employers, communities and even the medical personnel who
   see these black men when they report with
   other illnesses;

2. To give practical non-medical advice to the reader to take action to improve the prognosis and health;
3. To encourage black people, especially black men to own the issue of prostate cancer and realise that they play a huge role in reducing the number of people dying prematurely with the disease.

It is always good news when you hear or read that health outcomes in the United Kingdom, where I live, or wherever you live, continue to improve. People live longer than before; social conditions are getting better, and medical advances in technology have improved. There is no denying all of that. As a result, one would expect other aspects of life to be better. Yet, disparities in health outcomes for black men continue to exist.

Whether you are a black man, you know one, or you are a professional encountering black men in your daily work, I hope this book will give you a framework to work from and together we can increase awareness and promote better health outcomes for black men.

"No doubt cancer is not an easy subject to discuss, however, without discussion we will continue to perish."

Chapter 1
A Personal Mission

> *"If not me, who? And if not now, when?"*
> *~ Mikhail Gorbachev.*

I have become more interested in health issues as I grow older. Looking after my health and that of my family has become very important. I am a black man of African origin in my early 50s. I discovered and was astounded by the issue of prostate cancer in black men when I was pursuing my master's degree in public health at Nottingham Trent University in 2015. It precisely happened when I was looking for a topic to research on for my dissertation.

I came across few publications that talk about prostate cancer. What these publications were saying about **'prostate cancer and black men'** was the hook that made me build a close relationship with the subject.

I immediately knew that I found the right topic to focus on. However, not knowing much about prostate cancer I needed to research it further.

My initial reaction was that if black men had a higher risk of developing prostate cancer and the mortality rate was high;

What are the barriers to an early screening of prostate cancer in black men?

What is stopping the black men from seeking help?

What could be done to change the outcomes?

What kind of support is out there for black men?

What action is needed to encourage screening?

Who can be involved in making this happen?

As a black man, I had so many questions and felt it was my duty to research and raise awareness about this issue. It was not just about writing an academic paper anymore. There was much at stake. This became a personal mission, and I asked myself;

If not me, who? And if not now, when?"

Researching this would increase my knowledge on the subject and it would create an opportunity to share and educate others, and even contribute to saving or prolonging someone's life.

Anyway, I said to myself, *"this experience would make a huge difference in the world."*

I was confident that in the process, I would be able to meet and talk to people and raise awareness of the issue of prostate cancer in black men. I knew that, like me, there were many black men out there who did not know that we black men are at an increased risk of developing prostate cancer in our lifetime. For that reason, we need to be most vigilant in getting tested and seeking help because the cancer is curable, especially when detected at the earliest stages.

I felt that it was vital to investigate and identify the barriers and issues stopping us, black men, from getting screened. To have a better understanding of the issue of prostate cancer in black men, I used an empirical qualitative research method and read several and previous findings from other experts. This enabled me not only to identify the barriers but also to explore and gather the attitudes, behaviours, knowledge, experiences, and perspectives of black men about prostate cancer in general and screening, as well as the factors that influence their decisions to get screened or not.

I also interviewed more than 30 black men; some in a focus group and others as random individuals. I also made it my mission to bring it up in conversation with any black man I came across over a period of over two years. And this continues.

My interviews and general research have identified some barriers some of which included:

- a lack of knowledge of prostate cancer,
- problems with the way it is diagnosed (embarrassed about the procedure being invasive),
- health service systemic (i.e., not referring black men for screening . . .) and structural barriers (non-economic burdens or obstacles that make it difficult for black men to access prostate cancer screening . . . .),

More about the barriers to screening will be more discussed in chapter 5.

The discussion also provided some pointers as to the kind of intervention required to encourage black men to get screened and reduce morbidity and mortality.

Interestingly, when I was inquiring about the subject, I thought that the best place to check first before I started looking at the academic papers was to get in touch with some organisations well-known in the country for working to improve the care and welfare of those affected by cancer.

I contacted some organisations; however, the responses were astonishingly sparse. Despite the statistics, some organisations did not have much information on the risks and experiences related to black men and prostate cancer.

Other questions started to occupy my mind as I was reading and discovering more and more about the issue. It is easy to start blaming other people when you are right in the situation. In my case, I start thinking . . .

Is the situation somewhat unfair?

Is it preventable?

Black men should not have to die from this illness due to a lack of awareness, ignorance or any other egotistical or non-egotistical tendencies.

Initially, I thought; *"it is easy just to send all black men aged 40 and over to get screened to avoid unnecessary deaths."*

Obviously, it is not as easy as I thought. When you understand the system and its complexity, and the ways things work, you would know that it is not straightforward as it sounds. For instance, one day I went to see my doctor for something completely different. While I was there, I said to myself, why not ask the doctor if I could be screened or checked for prostate cancer.

After all, I fit the criteria of those who have the highest risk of developing the disease. I asked, and the doctor didn't think it was necessary to have me checked or screened for prostate cancer. She thought that I didn't seem to have any of the symptoms. That was it. I tried to explain; she wouldn't change her mind. One of the problems is right there. Much as I understand it, there are budget constraints and other issues. However, being a black man, in the high-risk category would have meant that maybe the doctor would take some interest.

Now imagine someone who is not as aware as I am, it would take them another 30 years to even think of asking for a test, by then, they would be in a much higher risk. This could easily be a put-off for some black men.

My Intervention and Engagement Blueprint

Writing this book is part of my Intervention and Engagement Blueprint. My mission is to ensure that as many people as possible are aware that black men have a higher risk of developing prostate cancer in their lifetime. At 1 in 4, while the statistics for the rest of the populations is 1 in 8, the odds are stacked against us.

More importantly, my greater aim is to help get as many black men as possible to know that early diagnosis significantly reduces the risk of premature death from the disease. That way they can make more informed decisions with the help of their loved ones.

The fear of the diagnosis label has a link with one's mental health and wellbeing. Ignoring the issue does not mean it goes away. We, black people need to know that there is a help; we also need to know that the situation will not improve if we don't all play our parts to raise more awareness, to encourage more screening, and therefore, improve the outcome for us black men.

However, no one community can tackle this issue on their own. This has to be a joint effort from all angles. I cover this in detail in chapter eight and chapter nine. The interventions need to happen at all levels; individual, interpersonal, community, organisational and policy levels; this is covered in chapter eight. The engagement must also take place in the different sections of society involving the women in our lives, the community, the religious leaders and the medical professional this is covered in chapter nine.

Writing this book is the first part of helping me to continue to fulfill my mission, and hope that the message will reach as many people as possible, but my work does not stop here. I aim to make the discussion about prostate cancer less stingy and more mainstream. I hope after reading this book, you will be convinced enough to join me and start making a difference and raising awareness in your way. Alternatively, you can contact me so that we can work together. The famous African proverb says; *"If you want to go quickly, go alone. If you want to go far, go together."*

I plan to join and help in the research, interventions, and engagement to increase diagnosis of prostate cancer in the black communities in the following ways:

1. Education in the community and religious settings to raise awareness about prostate cancer through running workshops and focus groups.
2. Work with mainstream organisations and policymakers to raise awareness of the struggles and barriers facing the black communities through seminars, lectures, and holding dialogues with the appropriate stakeholders.
3. Becoming the voice of Prostate Cancer campaign. I do not believe you can only make a difference if you have personally been diagnosed. I have never had prostate cancer, but I know I can take the lead and join the few black men championing the cause.

4. Continue to research ways in which black men can talk freely about general medical health and ways in which our female counterparts can help us to become more caring and very serious about this issue.

Your Challenge

Think of five ways in which you can make a difference in your community regarding prostate cancer today.

Chapter 2
What is Prostate Cancer

> *"Wisdom is wealth. Wisdom is like fire; people take it from others. If you close your eyes to facts, you will learn through accidents."*
>
> *~ Three African proverbs*

Prostate cancer is considered to be the most diagnosed and malignant cancer in the male population in the United Kingdom and the world over. Prostate Cancer is said to be malignant because it is capable of spreading into other and nearby organs and causing serious and, ultimately deadly damage, unless the cancer is carefully and adequately treated.

In the United Kingdom alone more than 40,000 new cases are identified yearly.

The mortality rate of blck men is 30% higher than in white men with a rate of 91.6 per 100,000. It is known that prostate cancer risk has increased in black men; however, deaths are not only affected by risk, but also by the treatment given.

Where is the Prostate and how Does it Become Cancerous?

The prostate is a small gland shaped like a walnut that is found only in men. It is situated between the penis and the bladder and surrounds the urethra. The prostate gland, of which core function is to contribute to the production of semen, becomes cancerous when it changes shape and size.

According to the statistics, around 47,300 people were diagnosed with prostate cancer in the UK in 2013, which amounts to around 130 cases a day. 54% of those diagnosed are 70 and over years of age. In the United Kingdom alone, nearly 11,300 men died of prostate cancer in 2014, which amounts to around 31 deaths a day or 13% of all cancer deaths.

What are the symptoms?

It might be useful to know some of the symptoms of prostate cancer. Now, I am not a medical doctor, and the information I am sharing in this book is based on my research from a public health point of view and my own experience as a black man.

I have compared and combined some sources and produce a more comprehensive list of the most commonly recognised prostate cancer symptoms. It is important to note that there are many good sources of information including the health services or other organisations in your country.

It is widely acknowledged that prostate cancer symptoms are not always obvious. The cancer grows slowly, and men can go on with their lives without noticing, feeling or recognising any of the symptoms.

In some cases, however, the cancer can grow much faster and requires urgent treatment before it spreads elsewhere outside the prostate gland. It is only when the cancer has progressed and spread that such symptoms could be felt. Some of the most known prostate cancer warning signs include:

Urinary symptoms of prostate cancer – Because of the prostate gland being close to the bladder and urethra, prostate cancer may be accompanied by a variety of urinary symptoms. Depending on the size and location, a tumour may press on and constrict the urethra, inhibiting the flow of urine. Some prostate cancer signs related to urination include:

- an increased need and frequency to urinate, mainly at nights;
- burning or pain during urination;
- having difficulty urinating or trouble to start and stop while urinating;
- loss of bladder control;
- decreased flow or velocity of urine stream;
- the feeling that the bladder has not emptied completely;
- the presence of blood in the urine.

Other prostate cancer signs and symptoms – Prostate cancer may spread to nearby tissues or bones. If the cancer spreads to the spine, it may press on the spinal nerves. Other prostate cancer symptoms include:

- blood in semen;
- difficulty getting an erection;
- painful ejaculation;
- swelling in legs or pelvic area;
- numbness or pain in the hips, legs or feet;
- bone pain that doesn't go away;
- the feeling of pain in the lower back or hips.

Unfortunately, since many men are not well aware of these symptoms, they can go on with life, thinking

WHAT IS PROSTATE CANCER • 15

that every discomfort or pain they experience is just part of the aging process. It might be something else. Until they have it checked; they will not know what it really is.

So, it is vitally important that men get screened at an early stage as it provides them with a bigger chance of being cured.

How is Prostate Cancer Diagnosed?

There are many ways of diagnosing prostate cancer. The most commonly and routinely used, include:

- measuring the amount of prostate cancer specific antigen (PSA) through blood test;
- conducting a digital rectal examination (DRE) during which a doctor feels the extent to which the prostate is changing in shape or feel; and
- conducting an ultrasound known as transrectal ultrasound (TRUS), which enables the collection, using a guided needle biopsy, of small fragments of the prostate.

What are the Risk Factors?

With regard to the risk factors, the likelihood of developing prostate cancer is dependent on many factors. The most widely accepted risk factors linked to prostate cancer include:

- Ethnicity – for instance, the risk of developing cancer in black men is much higher than white men. For black men the risk is 1 in 4, compared to 1 in 8 for white men;
- Family history – when you have a brother or father who had prostate cancer, the risk of developing the disease is high;
- Age – in general, the likelihood of developing prostate cancer is also associated with age. Men over the age of 50 are susceptible to develop the disease. However, when you are a black man aged 45 or over, you are advised to get screened as the risk is high; and
- Diet and lifestyle are also a risk. Physical activity and less fat in the diet are highly recommended to reduce the risks, although these apply to many other diseases.

How is Prostate Cancer Treated?

There are many different options for prostate cancer treatment. However, choosing a treatment is dependent on the stage of the cancer. Such treatment options include:

- Active surveillance which is concerned with observing the cancer closely and having regular examinations to quickly treat the cancer, should it show signs of progression;

- External beam radiotherapy which is concerned with using radiation to destroy the cancer cells;
- Radical prostatectomy is when surgery is conducted to remove the prostate gland;
- Hormone therapy involves preventing the production of the hormone testosterone which the cancer cells require to develop;
- Radiotherapy can also be used as another treatment option to treat both localised and advanced prostate cancer;
- Chemotherapy is also used to keep the cancer under control. It is concerned with slowing down the multiplication of the cancer cells; and
- Other treatments including Cryotherapy, High-Intensity Focused Ultrasound (HIFU), Antiandrogens may well be used, should other treatments be no longer effective.

What is the Survival Rate?

In America, the overall 5-year relative survival rate for prostate cancer among African Americans is 96%, compared to nearly 100% among whites. 91% of all prostate cancers among African

Americans are diagnosed at a local or regional stage, compared to 93% in whites; the 5-year relative survival rate for African Americans whose tumours are diagnosed at these early stages approaches 100%. Among African American men, the 5-year survival rate drops to 28% when the cancer has spread to distant sites compared to 27% in white men.

Although recent statistics show that, generally the survival rate picture is positive, it is important to note that this only applies to those who are diagnosed and follow treatment.

This positive picture is due to many reasons, the main of which include early diagnosis of the disease. For instance, the five-year survival rate becomes higher, almost 100 percent for white men compared to 96 percent for black men.

However, the picture for black men is different. If we consider the new research done by the George Washington University Cancer Centre in Washington DC, that African American have a gene that is likely to make the cancer more aggressive and drug-resistant, the survival rate for black men has to be different. This, according to the researchers, may be one of the causes of the large mortality disparity between black and white men

In general, there has been an improvement in policy in cancer services. Despite such progress and the commitment made by the UK government in 2011 to save 5000 lives every year and reduce inequalities in health in its strategy for cancer, the statistics still show that, 1 in 4 black men are still likely to have prostate cancer in their lifetime and that the survival rate remains low.

What is the Current Policy in Prostate Cancer?

Despite all the current statistics, no policy of mass screening is in place in the UK. Although there are programmes of mass screening in the United States, they use the PSA test to detect the Prostate Specific Antigen level in the blood. This screening method is considered by some to have poor specificity, and that high levels of PSA are not always associated with prostate cancer. Because of the poor specificity, the PSA test cannot be trusted enough to warrant a mass screening programme in the UK. According to Public Health England, high level of PSA in the blood can mean something else, although this is rare. In its Prostate Cancer Risk Management Programme advice to doctors, Public Health England points out that doctors should exercise their professional judgements and decide who should be tested regardless of whether they feel the symptoms or not.

However, there is an issue here. Some black men believe that doctors lack clear guidance from the government and the understanding that black men are at higher risk of having prostate cancer; and therefore, should always classified as a priority and referred for screening.

Despite these statistics, few black men know that their risk of developing prostate cancer is higher than the general male population. This already raises many questions about why this is the case and what needs to be done to increase and improve the level of awareness amongst the black male population. Although some hospitals start to refer black men for screening, it is always at a later stage, which reduces the chances of being cured; thus, lowers the survival rates for this group.

According to the Parliamentary Stakeholder Group in a briefing document published in 2012, the black male population in the UK experience inequalities in health outcomes. This is consolidated by the current statistics, but also by the higher mortality rate from prostate cancer amongst black men. It is argued that the mortality rate is 30 per cent higher than that of the white male population.

The consensus is that black men experience inequalities; whether intended or not is not the question. The question now is what can be done to increase awareness of prostate cancer and result in a better health outcome for black men?

In the United States and other parts of the world, the picture is no different. However, when the US Preventative Services Taskforce advised against prostate cancer screening, there was an overwhelming reaction against such decision, particularly, from the black community and health professionals alike.

This again brings the issue of inequalities to the forefront and asks the question why the black male population, since they are at higher risk of developing the disease, are not massively included in the study that led the US Preventative Services Taskforce to decide against prostate cancer screening. Being black is higher risk enough, in addition to other factors such as genetic, economic, education attainment and so forth.

Although not many studies have been conducted on the prevalence and morbidity rate of prostate cancer amongst the black male population in the United Kingdom, the few studies carried out seem to confirm what has already been done in the United States, and elsewhere.

They confirm that black men are at higher risk of having prostate cancer at a point in their lifetime than the white male population; and that the mortality rate for black men is 30 per cent higher than the white male population, which increases the likelihood of a black man dying from prostate cancer to over twofold.

The Importance and Benefits of Early Screening

The importance of screening or rather early screening increases the survival rate for prostate cancer patients. According to available studies the survival rate is dependent on how early the cancer is detected, provided that it is located in the prostate area only and has not spread to other areas or metastasised. Once it is spread, it is a whole new picture. For instance, in 2010 the National Cancer Registration and Analysis Service explained that in England between 1990 to 2002, the five-year survival rate amounted to over 90 per cent or more for localised cancer. For a metastasised cancer the rate was lower than 30 per cent.

According to Prostate Health UK, the latest information shows improvement regarding prostate cancer survival rate. For instance, if the one-year survival rate was around 65 per cent between 1971 and 1975, this trend has changed between 2004 and 2006 to amount 93 per cent and 94 percent between 2010 and 2011. About the five-year survival rate, research shows that for people screened between 2002 and 2006, the survival rate is 100 per cent if cancer has not spread outside the prostate area. Should the contrary happen, the survival rate is around 30 per cent. Once again this highlights the importance of early screening and how it affects the survival rates.

Prolonging life is the most important objective of prostate screening. To achieve that early diagnosis enables to deal with the cancer as early as possible and to prevent it from spreading to other areas, thus developing into what is known as symptomatic metastatic disease.

Amongst the benefits of early prostate cancer screening, according to Prostate Health UK, include:

- giving the early warning signs of prostate cancer before symptoms can be felt;
- detecting the cancer early when it could be cured;
- avoiding early death and prolonging life.

The Facts and the Reality

> *"Do not let what you cannot do tear from your hands what you can."*
> *~ Ashanti Tribe Proverb*

Inclusion and health inequalities are a reality that many health professional and communities deal with on a regular basis. Black men fall within the cohort of the population that have poor health outcomes. Meeting the health needs of this group of socially excluded individuals remains a challenge.

The black male population generally has poorer predicted health outcomes and a shorter life expectancy than the average comparable population. After extensive research and a lot of reading about prostate cancer, I found this to be true.

Several research publications have correlated the experiences of the black male population in relation to prostate cancer; that black men have higher risks of having prostate cancer than the white male population.

It is widely accepted that the incidence of prostate cancer in black men, including black men in their late 40s and 50s, is higher than any other cancer in the male population in general. Recent statistics show that the death rate for black men reached 30 per cent higher in comparison with that of the white male population and that the survival rate is dependent on whether prostate cancer was diagnosed at the earliest or latest stage.

I also discovered that prostate cancer is considered as the most threatening cancer to black men.

Research evidence shows that 1 in 4 black men is at more risk of having prostate cancer in their lifetime, compared to 1 in 8 white men. The statistics also reveal that the mortality rate is higher than that of other ethnic groups.

In addition to and despite the statistics, few black men know that they are at a higher risk of developing prostate cancer compared to the general male population. This disparity in itself raises many questions about why this is happening and what action needs to be taken to increase and improve the level of awareness amongst the black male population. Even though some hospitals take the initiative and start to send black men for screening, it is always in the late stages when the symptoms are already showing badly, which reduce the chances of being cured; thus, lowers the survival rates.

Chapter 3
Perceptions

Health Inequality

There have been many viewpoints as to the why and how health disparities exist between different sections of the society. Although several researches have been conducted over the years and have provided some of the answers, they do not highlight why such disparities still exist today.

One thing is clear though. It is widely known that the black male population health outcome is more negative than the white male population, in relation to prostate cancer. This situation is considered as unfair and preventable. This simply is referred to as health inequalities.

To have a better understanding of why a section of the society would experience such negative outcomes in their health for something that could be prevented or avoided is vital.

How does a situation like this manifest itself in society?

What does it have to do with prostate cancer?

The answer to such question is more complicated. However, I decided that it is worth revisiting the work of well-known academics and experts in the field of health inequalities. Perhaps I would find out something that explains why such situation happens in the 21st century. Many renowned academics have explored the issue to try to provide answers to similar questions. Some see health inequalities as being the systematic differences in the health of people occupying unequal positions in society and across social dimensions included income, social class, deprivation, cast, ethnicity, and geography.

In the process, they highlighted the importance of theorising health inequalities. They indicated that not only do health inequalities theories enable to identify the root causes of health inequalities, but also to devise better ways of tackling these causes.

One of the ground-breaking work into health inequalities was the Black Report published in 1980. The report concluded that health inequalities were caused by social inequalities in income, educational attainment, where people live, what they eat, employment or unemployment and conditions of work.

In addition to the Black report, some argue that cultural differences, the lack of understanding of the system could also contribute to the root causes of health inequalities.

The Black report was followed by others ground-breaking work into health inequalities in the UK including, the Acheson Report, the Marmot Review. All discussed the importance of reducing health inequalities and made many important and wide-ranging recommendations which influenced subsequent Governments' policies to this day in their endeavour to reduce health inequalities.

To understand how and why these health inequalities came about the Black Report suggests some theoretical explanations organised in 4 categories. These include what is known as:

- artefact;
- natural or social selection;
- materialist; and
- behavioural.

Regarding the **artefact** explanation of health inequalities, it is stated that this explanation rests on the idea that the relationship between class and health is artificial rather than real. It is a measurement phenomenon which arises either through the (inadequate) measurement of social class and health or in the measurement of the relationship between the two.

This means that the artefact explanation suggests that the relationship between class and health outcomes is a fabrication, although it is of historical and cultural interest. It has become the norm because of the way the class system was organised over a long period of time.

However, some people are critical of the theory, particularly when considering the overwhelming evidence of health inequalities around us. They believe that such theory is weak and of little significance.

Even when a different set of measurement is used, nobody can deny that the experience of black men, in relation to prostate cancer, has been different from that of white men. It is true; one can argue that not all black men are poor, illiterate and live in deprived areas.

However, the majority are. They might not be illiterate, but because of their ethnicity, and other circumstances, like not having the job that is equivalent to their experience and education, are condemned to do menial jobs and live in poor neighbourhoods. In general, if you are black, regardless of how successful you are; you are likely to be put in the same category as the so-called lower class.

The Black report explanation of the **natural or social selection** view of inequalities implies that those who are ill are automatically demoted to lower class; and those who are healthy are promoted to higher class.

This explanation presupposes that healthy lifestyle equals high social class, and poor health equals low social class. This means that this theory of selection suggests that this health characteristic can determine one's success and failure in life, and one's place in the social ladder. Considering the above explanation, chances are this could affect future generations' economic status, education, health and social mobility.

Furthermore, the selection view suggests that naturally, people tend to group themselves by their interests, ethnicity, gender, age, income, lifestyle, level of education. Whether it is the process of natural selection or not is a matter of interpretation. What is true is that social mobility can be encouraged by one's circumstances, be they economic, social, and educational and so on. This belief has been determining government policies for many years.

However, one cannot help noticing that such view seems to encourage more discrimination than eradicate it. It seems to reinforce the bigoted idea that when you are born disabled, for instance, your chances of succeeding in life and moving up the social class ladder are minimal.

So, what does this say about black men having prostate cancer?

Should we resign to the idea that if I am black and I have a higher risk of having prostate cancer; therefore, that is my fate and there is nothing I can do about it or I shouldn't do anything at all to improve the situation? I am doomed, that's it? This perhaps explains the fatalist attitude of black men in relation to prostate cancer.

The materialist or structural view put emphasis on one's socio-economic position. The more power and wealth you have the better chance you have to experience positive health outcomes.

That is to say that one's socioeconomic circumstances, including income and social capital, can determine one's health status and wellbeing. The physical environment is also important and can impact on health status.

Evidence shows that the experience of those living in deprived neighbourhoods is different from those living in affluent areas. For instance, poor neighbourhoods are known to have fewer, or sometimes nothing at all, leisure facilities, few green spaces, and a little encouragement towards a healthy lifestyle.

However, this structural view advances the idea that health inequalities can be tackled through economic means alone. It is true that this has a greater influence on people's health and wellbeing, but it is not the only factor that can be used to eradicate poverty and improve one's health and well-being.

It is unrealistic to think that, with the world wealth and power concentrated in the hands of the few, the powerful are going to give up their statuses to others under the pretext that they believe in equality, mainly when power and wealth are associated with better health.

The **behavioural view** is argued that this view supports the idea that the predominance of certain behaviours causes health inequalities. Such behaviours could include smoking, alcohol consumption, lack of exercise, diet and so on. The belief is that those in the lower part of the social ladder become unhealthy because they adopt unhealthy behaviours. They drink a lot, smoke a lot, eat unhealthy food, live a sedentary life, and so on.

The issue of health inequalities and its causes continues to be debated and researched, as Governments, other institutions, and communities are trying to find the way forward to address it and improve the health outcomes and well-being of all sections of the population.

It is important to note that the issues of health inequalities are paradoxical. Although the welfare state was created to minimise the impact of socioeconomic inequalities, inequalities in mortality and morbidity have increased. All the actions taken to tackle inequalities have not been sufficient enough; and to understand such paradox existing theories may help provide an explanation, knowing that socioeconomic inequalities come from social inequality.

In general, inequalities are said to exist as a consequence of the way society is stratified. Society is divided into classes. The most powerful belong to the upper class; the less powerful in the middle or lower classes, hence, the term social stratification.

This theory of Social stratification implies a system by which a society is categorised in hierarchy in relation to the people's levels of power, wealth and social standing. Those who have power, wealth or born in the high society are high in the hierarchy; and those who have less, or nothing are in the lower or lowest level in the hierarchy. Although it creates inequalities, social stratification is seen as one of the characteristic of society everywhere and cannot be avoided. It is universal and is passed over to generations. The reasons why social stratification exists is found in the following ideas, such as structural functionalism, social conflict, and symbolic interaction.

The Structural functionalism is concerned with the way society operates. Here inequality is accepted and is seen as playing an important part in the functioning of society, with each stratum or section of the society having a role and purpose.

The theory suggests that those who have important functions, like a surgeon who performs complex and more valuable procedures, are greatly rewarded; while those who do lower skill jobs, the kind of jobs anybody can do, their rewards are less. This is to say that the more people are rewarded – because of the importance and value of their jobs, not only do they earn a higher income, but also gain power – the more respect and social standing they get. The functionalist argues that this gain in power, high level of income, prestige and higher social standing motivates others to work hard.

However, social conflict theorists argue against social stratification as being impractical for the society, as they see it subsidising the more powerful to the detriment of the less powerful. The likes of Karl Max maintain that this kind of system has created class conflict because the two classes – the powerful minority and the oppressed majority – have nothing in common; and this is demonstrated in the unequal distribution of resources.

For them the system uses oppression and intimidation to bring the oppressed minority in line; thus, forces them, through the "superstructure" of society, such as political, and economic institutions, to agree to a consensus and accept the values, belief and principles of such society as decided and regulated by the ruling class.

According to the social conflict theorists, it is a matter of time before the oppressed working class realised that their economic and social conditions have deteriorated and rebel to ask for a change of the system.

Additionally, the symbolic interaction perspective is concerned with the particular and symbolic meaning or belief people have developed to interpret the world around them. Such belief, which dictates people's behaviours, manifests itself in people's interaction with others. This held belief also enables people to interpret others' behaviours, which overall creates a social bond. For instance, people tend to interact mainly with those who have or share the same social and economic status, lifestyle, educational and ethnic background with them. This is social stratification in practice. It is seen as inherent to all of us and categorises people together.

Symbolic interaction enables us to interpret people's identities and social experiences. Issues of race and gender are people's interpretation of what they believe to be true about people who look like them or not. This determines who to interact with and at what level.

However, the symbolic interaction theory misses the big picture of social interpretation. It creates inequalities and encourages discrimination in the cases of race and gender. This perspective would not account for social forces like systemic racism or gender discrimination, which strongly influence what we believe race and gender mean.

In relation to prostate cancer in black men, The Office of Minority Health in the United States expresses concern about the health negative outcomes experienced by black men, in general and also in prostate cancer. They argue that, despite the many attempts to address such inequality, the morbidity and mortality rates continue to increase.

It is suggested that tackling inequalities in prostate cancer requires innovative ways of doing things. *For instance, involving black men in prostate cancer research requires more efforts directed towards, mainly, identifying the reasons why black men suffer more from prostate cancer than other ethnic groups and how to redress such imbalance.*

In order to achieve this, I am of the view that black men, myself included, need to take the initiatives and start learning more about of prostate cancer screening and treatments. We must learn to avoid thinking of the screening experience as good or bad experiences.

In this context, the American Cancer Society proposes that education and screening should start much earlier for black men. This to ensure that by the time some reach the standard age of 45 their behaviours, attitudes, and perspectives would be moulded in such a way they would have a better understanding of the risks and know what they need to do.

In sum, health inequalities, as being usually employed, refer to the systematic differences in health status which exist between different population groups (e.g., different social classes or ethnic groups).

To have a better understanding of the reasons health inequality exist, health inequalities theorists argue that health inequalities are linked with the socioeconomic position of the population which derives from social inequality, which is a consequence of the way society is stratified. Society is divided into classes. The most powerful belong to the upper class; the less powerful in the middle or lower classes, hence, the term social stratification.

According to the health, inequalities approaches, people experience poor health outcomes because they are born in poor socioeconomic circumstances. People's unhealthy behaviours create health inequalities. Here, the issue of class is seen as fundamental in the approach. When one is ill, one is demoted to the lower position of the social ladder; and when one is healthy one goes up the social ladder.

Social stratification, which is considered a natural way of viewing the world around us, creates inequalities that are seen to be inherent in us. Our beliefs dictate our behaviours and influence how we determine who to associate or interact with.

The Health Belief Model

Regardless of people's socioeconomic circumstances or their positions in society, they must make health-related decisions. Several factors influence such decisions. To have a better understanding of these factors and how they influence individuals to make such decisions, in this case, to get screened for prostate cancer, the Health Belief Model has been relevant.

The Health Belief Model is a psychological model used to understand and predict health behaviours. It was first introduced in the 1950s by social psychologists Hochbaum, Rosenstock and Kegels who wanted to understand the factors that influence individuals to make a health-related decision.

The idea behind the Health Belief Model is that people are likely to take health-related actions, should they think that by doing so they can prevent negative health conditions. This means that individuals become aware of their susceptibility and acuteness to a health condition; the benefits of taking recommended health-related actions with confidence; and understand the barriers to taking action to promote healthy behaviours. Individuals are also likely to take action, motivated by cues or signals, i.e. information, the feeling of the symptoms, awareness events and so on.

The explanation of the model is relevant and can be used to have a better understanding of why and how people make the decision to be screened for prostate cancer and what influences them to do so. Such understanding is also crucial since it enables to better plan for a prostate cancer screening intervention.

The Health Belief Model asserts, that a person's action to get screened for prostate cancer, for instance is determined by that person understanding and belief that:

- they are at high risk to have the disease;
- the health problem is life-threatening, and
- by taking action, they increase their chances of prolonging their life or improving their quality of life.

When they understand that, for instance, the advantages of taking the decision to get screened are much greater than the disadvantages. Somehow a trigger may be needed to encourage the person to act.

Additionally, the Health Belief Model can be used to explain future health behaviours through examination of perceptions, attitudes, and beliefs. This is very relevant since its application has the potential to increase the screening of prostate cancer in black men.

The **Health Belief Model** as linked to prostate cancer has six concepts outlined as:

- Perceived Susceptibility;
- Perceived Severity;
- Perceived Benefits;

- Perceived Barriers;
- Cues to Action; and
- Self-Efficacy.

Perceived Susceptibility

The concept of perceived susceptibility presupposes the understanding of one's susceptibility to developing a health condition like prostate cancer in black men. It claims that when we black men believe that the risk of developing prostate cancer is high, this is likely to encourage us to take the decision to get screened.

Perceived Severity

Perceived Severity refers to the belief that if we black men understand the severity (high mortality rate in black men, low survival rate), of developing, let's say, prostate cancer; we will take action to prevent from dying from the disease.

This is crucial since we men, in this case, black men, in general, are reluctant to visit the doctor to seek medical help. It is always when our health situation has become worse when we take action. It can be too late at times. So, better understanding the effects of not being screened for prostate or being screened too late on ourselves, our

families and friends might be the trigger needed
to encourage us to make the right decision to get
screened.

Perceived Benefits

Perceived Benefits refers to the assumption that
if we understand the benefits of good health
behaviours or making decisions early, we will
take the relevant action to prevent the perceived
threat.

This means that, according to the Health
Belief Model, we will adopt health protecting
behaviours should we are convinced that such new
behaviours, like prostate cancer screening, will
either prevent the development of the disease or
enable the latter to be detected early to increase
the chance of being cured.

Perceived Barriers

Perceived Barriers mean that even though we
understand that a health condition is life-threatening and that taking the proper course of action will
reduce the perceived threat, barriers may prevent
us from taking such action. The perceived benefits must be greater than the perceived barriers to
enable the perceived barriers to be overcome and

new and positive behaviours adopted. Such barriers could include:

- costs for health insurance in the United States;
- perceived inconvenience;
- the fear of discovering that we have cancer and other diseases;
- the risk associated with making such decision (e.g., side effects of treatment);
- the belief that cancer cannot be cured; and
- discomfort (e.g., pain)

Cue to Action

Cue to Action could be a situation, people, and events that contribute to people adopting a new and more positive behaviour. Cue to action suggests that this view is a trigger for action. With the understanding of perceived susceptibility, barriers and benefits, the occurrence of an event can trigger action. Such cues could include:

- the feeling of the symptoms of prostate cancer;
- campaign to raise awareness;
- the death of a known person, relative or friend from prostate cancer, and so forth;
- a report or a documentary on TV; and so forth;
- attending a workshop or discussion on prostate cancer.

Additionally, another cue for action, for instance, was the presence of people who had prostate cancer during the focus group discussion. These people, who were willing to share their experiences, made some of us participants think twice before we vigorously argued against a diagnosis method (digital rectal examination) that will save our lives.

Self-Efficacy

Self-Efficacy is about our sense of confidence to adopt a preventative health behaviour like, for instance, the ability to take the initiative to go and get screened for prostate cancer.

In summary, the application of the Health Belief Model in this study has enabled me to explore and understand that black men have the potential to understand their susceptibility to prostate cancer and what could happen if they do not get screened. The model suggests that to be able to take action, an internal or external cue is important to trigger such action.

Chapter 4
Barriers to Screening

Before considering the barriers to prostate cancer screening in black men, I decided to explore the barriers to access health services for the black and minority ethnic (BME) population in general. In fact, this can provide relevant background information on the experiences of BME population whom the black male population is part of.

Available and recent studies have shown that we BME population have little knowledge of our health risks, which presupposes that we are likely to experience poor health literacy.

Presumptions and Structural Barriers

Additionally, the feeling of shame about our illnesses; the lack of trust of health professionals and systems; and the experience of racism led to us Black and Minority Ethnic population adopting some pessimistic views of the system and our health fate. Consequently, such attitudes have resulted in higher death rates, health inequalities, short life expectancy, and so on, amongst BME communities in general.

Although it has been widely recognised that we BME communities have over the years suffered poor health and negative health outcomes, and have experienced several barriers to using health and other services, it has been recently that this issue has been considered a health inequality issue, therefore, needs to be addressed.

This assertion is confirmed by many sources which maintain that the abovementioned barriers and other barriers including culture, language, faith or belief, as well as structural, are likely to affect the perception and use of services.

Other Determinants

BME communities are likely to be affected by or experience the following impediments:

1. They tend to live in poverty in deprived areas, and have experiences of racism and discrimination;

2. They are inclined to experience different lifestyles and cultures that make it difficult to access services;

3. They have little awareness of the services available to them; lack of understanding of hospital processes; have difficulties talking about personal health problems;

4. They tend to have little or no understanding of specific and high-risk diseases such as prostate cancer, diabetes, and heart diseases; this can be complicated by language barriers and literacy levels;

5. They have some different needs compared to the general population; and therefore, can be pigeonholed by health staff who lack cultural awareness and the ability to detect and understand symptoms of unfamiliar and non-European diseases; leading to experiencing institutional and locational barriers.

The lack of useful information and proper communication in different languages in the National Health Service Cancer services has, in some cases, been reported to be poor, which has been an issue experienced by black and minority ethnic communities.

All the barriers mentioned above and many others may have been the contributing factors that set the environment in which we black men are reluctant in using the services that are likely to help us prolong our lives and improve our quality of life. As a result, we black men are likely to experience similar disparities in our health outcomes unless such barriers are understood and overcome.

The statistics on the low participation in prostate cancer screening, low survival, and higher morbidity and mortality rates have prompted researchers to investigate further. The big question is; why we black men, who are likely to have prostate cancer at one point in our lifetime and die from it, are not getting screened to give ourselves the chance to live longer?

Because we black men get checked for prostate cancer at later stages than white men, it is crucial to look at the reasons behind our decisions to delay or avoid the screening of prostate cancer. It is worth exploring our belief systems, perceptions and experiences of prostate cancer.

Various studies have been carried out to try to identify the barriers to prostate cancer screening. Some of the emerging themes have been seen to be associated with:

1. personal and economic status;
2. socio-cultural environment and status;

3. religion or belief;
4. the physical environment where people live and work; educational attainment; and perceptions and expectations.

An investigation conducted in the United States, discovered that amongst the barriers to prostate cancer screening reported by black men include:

1. the lack of trust of healthcare professionals and the health system due to other people's past experiences;
2. the fear of discovering of and confirming the family history of prostate cancer, and a general fear of what next;
3. fear of the disease itself and the likelihood of complications and bad side effects emanating from the treatment;
4. the fear of death from prostate cancer (seen as a death sentence);
5. embarrassment or stigma and the fear of erectile dysfunction (losing one's virility);
6. the lack of cultural sensitivity from healthcare professionals;
7. costs, where insurance is needed;
8. poor or limited knowledge of the disease leading to a fatalist attitude (negative mindset and expectations of the health system);

9. the uneasiness of the diagnosis method known as Digital Rectal Exam;

10. the lack of role models from the black community that the community can look up to for motivation and encouragement;

11. the lack of communication with family and friends on their health issues;

12. age (the older one gets, the more motivated one is to get screened); and

13. black men are not taking the initiative themselves to go and get screened.

Similar studies, which show similar findings to those mentioned above, have identified amongst other barriers:

14. the fear of discovering other diseases during screening;

15. not having a regular doctor;

16. the lack of courage and unwillingness to see a doctor;

17. the lack of understanding of the importance of disease prevention.

These barriers have also been confirmed by the focus group interview discussion and some of the individuals I talked to during the research. Although all of the black men participants showed some level of awareness of prostate cancer, they were not aware of:

1. the statistics;
2. the symptoms;
3. how it is diagnosed;
4. the higher risks associated with us black men;
5. the importance and benefits of early screening;
6. the disparities in health outcome for us black men due to the identified barriers and other factors.

Perhaps the presence of some of the participants who either had prostate cancer or on treatment for prostate cancer has energised the discussion and given the impression that almost everyone had some level of understanding of what prostate cancer was. Some of the participants commented that the basic knowledge is out there and is accessible to everyone.

Yet, most of the people I talked to had little or no knowledge about prostate cancer and the risk factors associated with black men.

This is why, considering the statistics and the seriousness of the issue, I am convinced that many more discussions like this between ourselves as black men or black communities are needed everywhere. These will galvanise and encourage us to look deep into ourselves and realise that we need to change to be able to take care of ourselves and live longer.

From my experience of speaking to many of my brethren and observation, I think the main barrier for us black men to get screened for prostate cancer is deep-seated in our behaviours, attitudes, and ways of thinking towards the disease and to health in general.

For instance, **I was somewhat surprised by the reaction of the majority of the black men present in the focus group discussion against the Digital Rectal Exam, one of the main methods used to diagnose prostate cancer. Almost everyone had a negative view of this method.** They felt that it would be an invasion of their privacy and masculinity, and it was something that some would find difficult to do.

This may have something to do with the cultural and traditional teachings about what is right or wrong about sex and sexual experiences. In most cultures, sexual practices such as oral sex and anal sex are frowned upon and seen as a taboo. Education and intercultural marriages and sexual relationships have led to some personal acceptance of such practices. However, there is still a high level of discomfort with the thought of a stranger (medical professional) having access to the private areas. This is especially so for men. Women have many opportunities to get examined or open up to non-sexual partners, making them more at ease with having similar examinations.

The folklore on a man's private parts in many African communities is a matter of great pride. There are several beliefs and competitiveness that men have to live up to. Some men would vow to die than have someone examine their private areas.

In sum, this book has identified some barriers that stop us black men from taking the initiative to get screened for prostate cancer. Some of these barriers can be overcome, should we black men gather the courage and willingness to do what is right for ourselves and our families; in addition to other support, including advice, education, family, friends, communities, health professionals, and policymakers.

Chapter 5
The Taboo Subject

> "*You learn how to cut down trees by*
> *cutting them down.*"
> *- Bateke Tribe proverb*

You learn how to cut through beliefs by educating yourself to cut through them. There is a common belief and acceptance that we black men don't like talking about our health issues. These beliefs can be deeply engrained in people's minds because in the cultural upbringing. Talking about certain subjects are seen as taboos.

Taboos, understood as unwritten laws restraining people from breaking social norms, were used to preserve harmony in the society and the good relationship with spiritual beings. Since a good life was dependent on harmony within society, anything disturbing it, such as unexpected death, sickness, disaster could be interpreted as resulting from breaking of some moral laws, especially taboos.

Certain diseases such as cancer were unexplainable and often seen as someone may have done something that breaks the taboo. The lack of knowledge about cancer and the causes is one of those difficult issues to talk about. Some people who are more on the religious side believe that suffering certain illnesses is a punishment from God. An alternative belief is that whatever happens to one is God's wish hence no reason to tempt fate. The outcome will be the same whether or not one gets checked. If you were meant to die you will die regardless.

Mentioning The 'C' Word

Even without having any preconceived ideas, it did not come as a surprise in my research to find that most of the black men I spoke with had reservations about mentioning the so-called 'C' word (cancer). There is a superstitious belief that talking about prostate cancer would bring about bad omen or you would be casting an evil spell on yourself.

During the focus group discussion, one participant commented; *"it is taboo to talk about these things."* Meaning talking about male sexuality and men's private parts and illnesses relating to them was taboo. He could not even bring himself to mention the words prostate cancer. This was followed by agreement from most members of the focus group. The disease is still widely regarded as a taboo subject within many families and in the black community.

Talking about one's health problems is considered as a sign of weakness. Instead of talking about our health issues and seeking professional help, we black men are frequently told to 'pray it away' or to 'man up and stop being feeble.' This is particularly prevalent in the older generations.

Religious Beliefs

The majority of the black men in the discussion are religious and derived strength from their spiritual beliefs. In times of emotional or physical difficulties, they reported that they turned to their religious belief as a coping mechanism. Certainly, many of the groups stated that if you leave things in God's hands only, He can find solutions.

There is nothing wrong there. However, for me, this is a misinterpretation of their belief. God will help when one takes the initiative to do something about it. One can pray to ask God to increase one's faith whatever the outcome, for the strength to do the right thing, God will not arrange to see and talk to your doctor for you.

God understands our weaknesses as humans and can see through us. One would think it is the religion speaking, but in fact it could be that the fear of finding out the problem is what is stopping us black men from getting examined for prostate cancer. I believe that by getting the examination earlier, we would find the problem sooner which would save our lives.

All religion promotes good health and wellbeing. By using religion not to seek help we merely confirm what is next, fear. Fear takes over our thoughts and, in some cases, there might not be anything to worry about. As they say: "help yourself, and God will help you."

Some of the participants in the focus group discussion expressed their concerns, particularly when they learnt about what the statistics said about prostate cancer in black men. They believed that considering these statistics and other factors; we black men should automatically be referred for screening; something the doctor does not always do.

Kwame, one of the participants, related a story about someone he knew and who did not survive prostate cancer; because when he was diagnosed the cancer had already spread to other areas. He then reiterated the fact that we black men should always be referred by our doctors for screening. Participants believed that Public Health organisations, the Health Services, Chief Medical Officers, the Department or Ministry of Health should issue a guideline to all health centres or clinics that guarantee that we black men aged 40 and over are automatically referred for screening for prostate cancer. This should be the national policy.

Some of the black men I spoke to believe that prostate cancer campaigns lack role models from the black community to engage with and encourage black men to get screened. They believe that such role models may make a huge difference, in terms of communicating the prostate cancer risk factors associated with being a black man and the benefits of getting screened early before it is too late. Perhaps they could help break our taboos.

So how can we encourage more role models?

What do we need to do to get more people talking about prostate cancer?

How can we stop this disease from claiming more lives?

There is no single answer to these questions. However, we can take steps towards ensuring we are well aware of the prostate cancer threat and take action to change our lives for the better and the statistics. None of us want to be a statistic. Some answers to these questions are provided in the next chapter where I talk about the kind of intervention needed and which role we must play to change the situation.

As Amari, one of the participants put it: *"we should have more adverts on TV, we black men need to change our mindsets when it comes to prostate cancer."* During the discussion, we all agreed that, other than talking to our doctors, we were not well aware of any other available support systems.

We did not have any idea of what to do should we feel some of the symptoms or just wanted to talk about the issue or have a specific question. No one in the group knew what they needed to do if they wanted to talk about worries and fears of prostate cancer. In addition to men taking the matters seriously and taking action, I also believe women need to get involved in the campaigns too. The men are co-conspirators, and the women in our lives are protagonists. They have the ability to influence and persuade men to get examined.

One participant Ayomide, who is a prostate cancer survivor said that people should not fear to get checked. What matters is that people have the chance to prolong their lives by leaving fear aside and get screened regardless of the method used. Although, as he put it, he understood the reluctance of black men to get checked, he explained that anybody who cared about themselves and their families should get screened.

Remember as Joyce Meyer puts it, *"I believe that the greatest gift you can give your family and the world is a healthy you."*

So, what kind of interventions do we need to tackle the identified barriers and improve awareness and change our behaviours, attitudes, perceptions, and assumptions regarding prostate cancer? What role can every one of us play?

There have been many suggestions on the best way to tackle the barriers stopping us black men from getting screened for prostate cancer, and the disparities in our health outcomes we have experienced.

For instance, the participants in the focus group came up with many ideas on how we could improve awareness and encourage ourselves to get screened. Some believe that the lack of organised events like the focus group discussion when we as a community could be consulted on the best way forward to educate and encourage ourselves to get screened can constitute a barrier to prostate cancer screening. Therefore, we were unanimous in suggesting that a mass campaign needs to be carried out, mainly where black communities were largely present.

I understand these taboos we mentioned earlier exist and are entrenched in the culture. No matter how educated or progressive we are, these ways of thinking seem to get the upper hand at times. Who cares if a doctor put his/her finger in the backside so long as it saves my life and that I will be around my loved ones for a long time? We make as if this kind of procedure takes forever. It might only take few seconds or minutes to check the prostate.

Does it really matter what procedure is being used?

Another point, I think it is high time we stopped these taboos getting in the way of important and life and death decisions. I think we have reached a point in human development that we understand that some taboos do not make sense. We have to be open and confident to talk about our health issues, worries, and fears. It can only help us overcome them.

Embarrassment

Would you rather die of embarrassment or ignorance?

Is it not better to stay alive for ourselves and for those who love us?

Don't get me wrong! I am not saying that it is an easy thing to do. But as long as we can start, the rest can follow. It will take time to change our way of thinking. This goes with the way of thinking which we need to change. Talking to our partners, for instance, about health issues, our worries and fears can only help us. It is a good start to start rallying support, God forbid, should something unexpected were to happen.

I understand many have found the statistics shocking and couldn't believe what they had just heard. Even more than the shock, it is more worrying that in 2017, with all the adverts on television and other media about cancer, the level of knowledge was surprisingly low.

"Very few men and women had an understanding of the symptoms, what to do, where to go and who to talk to."

One day I had a conversation with a young man who I will call Tunde. He was a very well-educated young man and had been married for three years. We talked about many aspects of life as a black man in the UK and life in general. He was very knowledgeable, but one thing still stood out for me, he told me: *"I never thought about me having prostate cancer. It is not something black men talk about. In general, we black men we are very bad at talking about our health issues. So, now I am a bit aware of the statistics, if I want to get checked, what do I do?"*

My answer to the above question was that if he wanted to discuss the issue and the possibility of getting checked, he needed to talk to his doctor who would advise him of what to do. I also told him that he could contact Prostate Cancer UK; they might give him some further information and insight about prostate cancer.

Another thing Tunde could do is to talk to his partner about prostate cancer in black men. He might get the encouragement he needs from his partner to go to talk to his doctor. His partner might even suggest going with him to the doctor for support and confidence. The more we talk about it, the more we feel confident enough to go through with it.

During the focus group discussion, the few theme that emerged was methods of diagnosis (DRE), lack of role model from the black community, the lack of effective awareness in the black community, knowledge of prostate cancer and available support systems, access to screening services, culture, communication and personal responsibilities and intention to get screened.

One of the main points of discussions was one of the diagnosis methods known as the Digital Rectal Exam (DRE), commonly used to detect prostate cancer. It appeared in the conversation that some were very concerned about and strongly against the DRE method of diagnosing prostate cancer.

Kofi aged around 40-45 said: *"This can be construed as a cultural thing in the black community. This physical thing with the finger in the backside. It is considered as an invasion of privacy and the black man masculinity"*. Another black man, Jabulani added: *"Oh no! No doctor put his finger in my backside"*. Everybody started laughing. *"This is very serious,"* added Yohannas, looking a bit annoyed, as the others were laughing off.

However, one of the older men, Thenga, who had just recovered from prostate cancer added: *"I understand your concern and the attitude of black men in general; but what is important? To save your lives? I think it is time you black men started to take responsibility for yourselves and your health.*

If I did not get checked earlier, I would have been a dead statistics by know. I am glad they put their finger in my backside because I am alive right now. You might be young and think you are immune. But as you've just heard the statistics, most of you are likely to have prostate cancer. It is harsh, but you have to listen.

I have just recovered from prostate cancer; other friends did not. I am lucky, and I thank God for it every day. If my doctor did not refer me for screening, I wouldn't be here by now. It was difficult for me, for my family, my children, and grandchildren and my friends. But we all come together and support each other. You will need your family around you should the worse were to happen. God forbid".

I believe the presence of 2 older black men who experienced prostate cancer in the focus group had increased the interest of the participants and the desire to look after their health. The presence of the prostate cancer survivors in the discussion who were willing to share their experiences, made some of the participants think twice before they laughed off and vigorously argued against a diagnosis method that will save their lives.

Another point of discussion was around the type of interventions that would help raise awareness of prostate cancer and tackle the barriers to screening. Almost all participants in the focus group agreed that the involvement of a role model is key to increase awareness and screening.

Abiola, one of the participants, added: "*we have to ensure we have a role model from the black community who can act as a prostate cancer ambassador. Someone who is in the public eye and seen as trustworthy that the community can look up to. Perhaps this will encourage black individuals to go and get checked".*

Khamari, another participant stated that communication was another important issue. He added: *"although awareness raising adverts and events were happening in the country, these were not reaching the black community. I am a prostate cancer survivor, and when I went to the hospital for my check-up and treatment, I only saw white men, as I was waiting to see the doctor. If I was not already diagnosed I would have said; It's only for white men. So, the solution would be to have a targeted and intensive campaign for the black community, using famous role models who would carry the message to the community. The few advertisements on television do not have many black people, if at all, in them. Because of the statistics, this is the right thing to do".*

Another participant was concerned about the cost of such campaign. He pointed out: *"who pays for it?"*

There was an assumption that in the UK not much has been conducted or researched to ensure that black men have access to health services. There have been few organisations and individuals in the

community that were involved in taking the prostate cancer message to those at more risk, such
as the black male population. However, it is still
not enough to motivate black men to get screened
because of the barriers some of which are personal,
cultural, systemic, socioeconomic, and political.

They were not aware of the statistics that show
disparities in health outcome for black men due to
the identified barriers and other factors.

Superstition

Additionally, many argue that black men don't
like talking about their health issues. There was a
superstition that is talking about it would enhance
its malevolent power. Nzingha, one of the participants commented that:

> *"most black people don't like to talk about . . .
> that they have got cancer. They just see it as a
> taboo; in fact, I know a lot of people who do not
> even mention the word".*

Furthermore, Tambia argued that people should not
fear to get checked. What mattered was that people
would have the chance to prolong their lives by
leaving fear aside and get screened regardless of the

method used. Although he understood the reluctance of black men to get checked, he explained that anybody who cared about themselves and their family should get screened. *"It was a daunting prospect to think that my family was suffering as well as I was and that I was not going to be around to take care of them."*

The discussions we had have been useful. I believe all the black people I talked to, one way or another, took something away with them. The discussion has also provided some level of understanding of black men's attitudes, perspectives, beliefs, and experiences towards prostate cancer. I would like to see discussions like these taking place everywhere to enable black men to talk about health issues, mainly prostate cancer. The next stage of my mission is to ensure discussions are taking place everywhere to mobilise and motivate black people, increase black men's confidence to tackle health issues, to tackle barriers, to break taboos, to put pressure on policy or decision makers to do something to facilitate access to the relevant service and support.

Aside from taboos and other beliefs, fear is a huge underlying issue affecting many of us. Cancer is not an easy disease to deal with. We need to be brave and make the right decision for us and our loved ones.

> *"The brave man is not he who doesn't feel afraid, but he who conquers that fear."*
> ~ **African Proverb**

Chapter 7
Interventions

> "*Sticks in a bundle are unbreakable.*
> *It takes a village to raise a child.*"
> ~ *African proverbs*

Intervening to increase awareness and confidence is about trying to change the behaviours, attitudes, beliefs, and perspectives of the black male population about their health, in general, but more importantly about prostate cancer. Not only does this require devising effective and innovative tools or methods to communicate an already existing message, but also to learn to understand these characteristics that need changing.

There are many ways to educate us black men and to raise awareness and improve the uptake of prostate cancer screening. Over the last few years, few and limited campaigns have been devised. Some have worked; some have not. This explains the lack of knowledge of prostate cancer from many black men. Awareness education on prostate cancer is important; however, it depends on how it is transmitted, who transmits it. Personalised intervention is key to change and influence behaviour.

It is important to note that there are different levels of intervention to increase awareness and address the barriers to prostate cancer screening in black men. These do not stop at individual or community level. They go further than that.

It is also important to have the pledge of policy makers, health institutions, and organisations, health professionals, communities, families, religious and community leaders. Each section has a specific role to play, and at the same time, all work together to achieve a common objective, which is to increase screening of prostate and prolong the lives of black men.

It is crucial since it enables to create a suitable and positive environment and facilitate the processes and procedures in the screening of prostate cancer. In order to have a very successful intervention, I suggest the following model, the **Intervention and Engagement Model**. The model illustrates the levels and roles of each section in the fight against prostate cancer in black men. It suggests what can be done and how. This model is inspired and adapted from the Unicef Social Ecological Model & Communication for Development Method

Intervention and Engagement Model

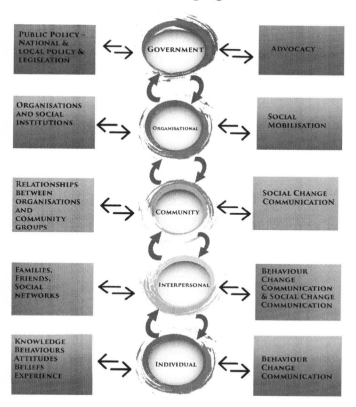

Description of Intervention and Engagement Model

This model illustrates the importance of adopting a multidisciplinary approach to increasing awareness and screening of and preventing prostate cancer, as well as addressing the barriers and disparities experienced by us black men. The model highlights the importance of the levels of influence, with each level playing its part, and at the same time working with other levels to bring about a more positive outcome and impact.

The focal point of the model is the individual, the black man, supported by four levels of influence including the interpersonal, organisational, community, and government or policy levels.

The model shows how the levels are interlinked, and that no one level can do the work alone. Any public health initiatives need to involve and be implemented at these five levels to guarantee maximum synergies of intervention for maximum impact.

In sum, the essence of this intervention and engagement model is in its multidisciplinary approach, as it focuses on recognising the importance of the relationships and interactions between these levels of influence on health and health behaviours. These levels of influence are outlined below.

Individual Level

The characteristics that influence black men behaviour change and shape positive health behaviours, including knowledge, attitudes, behaviour, self-efficacy, beliefs, gender, age, ethnicity, sexual orientation, economic status, trust, expectations, education, fear and so on.

At this level the main objective is to increase the black man's knowledge and influence his behaviour, attitudes, beliefs, and experience towards:

- The need to be screened for prostate cancer
- The intention to be screened or tested for prostate cancer
- Understanding the risks and benefits of screening for prostate cancer.
- Accessing effective and convenient prostate cancer screening, diagnosis, and treatment.

The model shows that, for any prostate cancer screening initiatives, the black man is the focal point. It highlights the importance of increasing awareness of prostate cancer to educate the black male population of the risks and benefits of screening, as well ensuring that timely, appropriate and high-quality prostate cancer screening treatment is provided to the individual who is diagnosed with cancer.

Interpersonal Level

Social networks and social support that influence black men behaviour, including family, colleagues, friends, and so on.

The model shows that at this level numerous prostate cancer prevention and awareness-raising activities are taking place. These activities are intentional and should be aimed at encouraging change in the black man's behaviour and overcoming social and cultural barriers. Here, family, friends, social networks, health care professionals, health trainers, patient representative groups, community health workers, colleagues, etc. are key in the relationship. They carry a message of support to and remind the black man that he is not alone in this journey. They are part of several interventions, including:

- Doctors, advising and making referrals for prostate cancer screening;
- Black men being reminded of the need to be screened by friends, family, etc.; and
- Patient representative groups, friends, and family help remove and overcome barriers to screening (e.g., fear . . .).

Community Level

Community groups, associations or forums, neighbourhoods, community and religious leaders, businesses, people, schools, etc. and their formal or informal relationships among themselves and with organisations, institutions, and other networks within defined interests, boundaries, rules and social norms – working together for the betterment and wellbeing of communities.

At this level, the model shows that prevention activities are important and need to be implemented at the community level. Like at the interpersonal level, these activities are intentional and are aimed at encouraging change in black man's behaviour. The difference to the interpersonal level is that more resources from community-level organisations or groups – e.g., community & voluntary sector organisation are deployed. Such community-level organisations or groups might include local health and wellbeing partnerships, the media, community advocacy groups, etc. Interventions activities at this level could include:

- Working in partnership and collaborating with community-level groups to promote prostate cancer screening;
- Organising and carrying out influential public awareness and educational campaigns;
- Organising at the grassroots level to influence the relevant authorities and change the status quo; and

- Collaborating with health departments to develop a mass screening for prostate cancer.

Organisational Level

Organisations, civil society organisations, health organisations – health services, hospitals, and clinics, commissioning groups, public health organisations, prostate cancer organisations, etc. – and processes that influence health behaviours, as well affect how effective services are provided to black men.

At this level, the intended activities to encourage individual behaviour change should aim at ensuring that organisations – healthcare systems, doctor surgeries, health services, hospitals, health clinics, employers, etc. – have systems, practices, and policies in place that influence the effectiveness of the services provided to black men. Many experts interact at this level. Their advice is potential sources of organisational messages and support. Examples of interventions for this level include:

- Sending out regular invitations and reminders to black men for prostate cancer screening;
- Yearly check-ups for over 40 black men to automatically offer to conduct a prostate cancer examination;

- Putting in place assessment and feedback systems to measure performance on encouraging positive health behaviour;
- Promoting the benefits of prostate cancer screening; and
- Adopting workplace policies that encourage employees to take positive health decisions, i.e., prostate cancer screening.

Policy Level

Laws, policies, and practices at the local, county, regional, national and international levels that promote or regulate health behaviour. This could include the deployment of resources.

At this level, activities include enacting legislation and policies that facilitate prostate cancer screening for the black male population. Activities also include interpreting and implementing existing policy and legislation. Political parties, local councils, regional and national agencies may support policies that promote positive, healthy behaviour, including screening for prostate cancer. Examples of activities include:

- Health department working in collaboration with other government departments and other institutions to communicate prostate cancer screening policy to the public, and to tackle the barriers to screening and the existing health disparities in black men;

- Health services, public health agencies and other agencies producing clear guidance on prostate cancer screening, placing black men as a priority.

Chapter 7
The Engagement Approach

The engagement approach, as part of the Intervention and Engagement model, is used to engage the five level of influence – individuals, communities, organisations, professionals, policymakers – at local and national levels, in a dialogue towards advocating for the development and implementation of policies and programmes that reduce health inequalities and promote good health and wellbeing for the black male population, with a particular focus on prostate cancer. The Intervention and Engagement Model will not be complete without the Engagement Approach.

The engagement approach also aims to empower and strengthen the capacity of communities, so that they are able to:

- advocate for the health issues affecting their communities,
- influence behaviour changes in individuals and policy at local and national levels.
- facilitate dialogues and collaborations with influential groups

Below are a presentation and description of the engagement approach. It is important to note that each proposed action corresponds to a specific level of influence in the Intervention and Engagement model. However, some proposed actions can be applied to other levels of influence. For instance, advocacy can be used at different levels.

Summary of the Engagement approach

Proposed Actions	Intervention activities	Actors
Advocacy	• Aims at influencing the development and implementation of effective legislation, policies, and practices	• Policy makers and government officials • Community groups • Community leaders

Proposed Actions	Intervention activities	Actors
	• Focuses on mobilising communities around a health issue, and uses evidence message to encourage a programme of actions	• Patients reference groups • Equality groups
Social Mobilisation	• Aims at building a strong partnership at the national and community levels for a common purpose • Focuses on communities' empowerment and building a collective force that can influence change at all levels • Focuses on facilitating dialogue, building a coalition, community groups or organisational activities	• Community leaders • Community groups or organisations • Public and private partners • Role models
Social Change Communication	• Focuses on encouraging individuals to engage in the process to help define their needs, advocate for their rights, and collaborate to change their social system	• Groups of individuals in communities • Role models

(Continue)

Proposed Actions	Intervention activities	Actors
	• Focuses on encouraging dialogue to change behaviour on a large scale, including social and cultural norms, and address inequalities • Focuses on progressively building interpersonal communication, community dialogue, mass & social media campaigns	
Behaviour Change Communication	• Focuses on building individual knowledge and skill; changing attitudes and behaviour; improving self-efficacy; increasing motivations • Focuses on progressively building interpersonal communication, community dialogue, mass & social media campaigns	• Individuals • Families • Partners • Women support groups • Friends • Colleagues • Men support groups

Advocacy

The government or policy level of the Intervention and Engagement Model is the platform where many major decisions – policy, legislation, guidance, practices, and funding that impact on the health of the population – are made. To influence the leadership at this level and other levels to take the appropriate course of action to improve and sustain the health of the population, a great support is needed from the public. In this case, advocacy is the process and effort to inform and motivate the leadership to create the appropriate environment for achieving positive health outcomes for all sections of the society. Advocacy aims to:

- promote the creation of new and fit for purpose policies, laws and practices; improve existing ones and ensure these are properly translated, impact assessed and implemented;
- influence the deployment of resources for specific initiatives aimed at improving and protecting the health of the population;
- influence governments at all levels to come up with appropriate programmes aimed at increasing awareness, increasing and facilitating prostate cancer examination for black men.

The following are examples of types of advocacy:

- ***Community advocacy*** – to empower communities to have their voices heard on issues that are important to them; call for change in policy, priorities, laws, practices, guidance, etc.

- *Policy advocacy* – to influence the government or policy makers or decision makers to come up with the necessary policies, laws, and practices that tackle health inequalities; improve and protect the health of the population; and facilitate equal access to health services (i.e., screening, treatment and aftercare services).

- *Media advocacy* – to involve all types of media to push the government or policy makers or decision makers to do more to help the most disadvantaged sections of the society.

In sum, advocacy is about influencing or motivating the government, or policymakers or decision makers to do something about an important issue that affects society or sections of the society; such as enacting new policies and practices, committing resources to improve a particular situation.

Social Mobilisation

Social mobilisation refers to the actions taken to engage and motivate various intersectoral partners at national and local levels to raise awareness of a particular issue, and advocate for a change in policy, laws, practices, etc. to tackle such issue.

Such partners could involve:

- the government or policy makers or decision makers,
- community leaders,
- health professional groups,
- religious leaders or groups,
- community and voluntary sector organisations,
- private sector organisations,
- community groups,
- individuals and influential role models.

This engagement approach focuses on people and communities as agents of their own change. It emphasises on:

- empowering communities,
- creating an enabling environment for change, and
- helping build the capacity of the groups involved in the process, so that they are able to mobilise resources, plan, implement and monitor activities with the community.

Other channels and activities for social mobilisation could involve:

- mass media awareness-raising campaigns,
- advocacy with community leaders to increase their commitment to the issue, and activities

that promote broad social dialogue about the issues, such as talk shows on national television and radio, community meetings, traditional newspapers, and leaflets. The idea is to ensure there is a strong and supportive environment that enables to empower communities to take action at the grassroots level.

Here, the black communities need to come together as a force of influence, not only to educate the black male population of the threat posed by prostate cancer but also of the benefits of getting screened as early as possible.

Social Change Communication

Social change communication refers to the intended process that creates the environment for groups of individuals or communities to identify and voice their needs and work together with others to bring about change. For instance, such process will empower black individuals or groups and put them in positions where they are able to change black men behaviours on a large scale, and tackle health inequalities.

The idea here is to ensure that individuals and communities are empowered and take ownership of such mobilisation with the collaboration of other key players.

Engagement activities and channels could include:

- social media;
- television and radio;
- communities and cultural events information distribution;
- presentations in community events;
- community-led presentations at parliaments, council or city assemblies, schools, etc.

Behaviour Change Communication

Behaviour change communication aims to promote positive health outcomes. It refers to an interactive process that enables to create a message specific for the black male population, using a targeted approach solely for this population. The objective of such specific and targeted message is to encourage change in knowledge, attitudes, and behaviours at individual and community levels, using black communities' communication channels.

The behaviour change communication approach will be a useful approach to:

- raising awareness and encouraging serious community discussions about prostate cancer in black men and related issues;

- increasing knowledge about prostate cancer and the benefits of getting screened;
- encouraging change in attitude, behaviour, and belief towards prostate cancer and the risks associated with not taking the initiative to get screened;
- fighting against any perceived community taboos that stop black men from talking about their health issues and seeking the appropriate medical help before it is too late;
- voicing strongly the issue of prostate cancer in black men to the government or policy makers and health services leaders to ensure they take notice of the issue and work to reduce the high mortality and increase the low survival rates of black men; and
- promoting and establishing services, specifically for advising black men and their families on prostate cancer prevention measures and management.

It is important to note that for the engagement model to produce the maximum and desired effects, these approaches – advocacy, social mobilisation, social change communication, and behaviour change communication – need to be combined since they are interdependent and interactive. For instance, the advocacy approach can be used to bring about new policies or change existing ones, new laws, and practices that will help facilitate change. A multidisciplinary approach is key to change social, cultural, or institutional norms and create the environment for behaviour change.

Health Professionals

Health services and public health organisations should ensure that health professionals are properly trained and are aware of the issue of prostate cancer in black men. They should ensure that, through their advice, a proper guidance is produced. Such guidance should facilitate access to health services and screening and highlight the priority given to prostate cancer in black men. Doctors should be able to refer any black man, aged 40 and over for screening. Health professionals should also be aware of the cultural sensitivities as this is likely to help them in the planning of educational and awareness schemes and screening in the community.

Some people are concerned that the messages put across in the media and reports seem to focus on the gory details or fear. The result in some black men tends to blank it out and avoid getting tested.

We must emphasise that symptoms similar to prostate cancer also appear in diseases that are not cancer-related, and that the treatment for prostate cancer is usually straightforward. A balance should be sought, between ensuring that men are motivated to pay attention to their health, without making them shy away from it because of fear. In the era of internet availability, it is important not to lead these men into self-diagnosis via the internet.

Health professionals must ensure that more reassuring messages are being put out on the internet. This can be achieved through targeted case studies, through blogs, adverts, magazines and men's clubs

Policy Makers

It is important to note that there are different levels of intervention to increase awareness and address the barriers. These do not stop at individual and community levels. It is important to have the pledge of policy makers and health professionals. This is crucial since it enables to create a suitable and positive environment and facilitate the processes and procedures in the screening of prostate cancer.

The government has the power to enact or improve existing laws, policies, and guidance and practices that facilitate intervention and engagement. It can also provide funding to pay for a national awareness-raising campaign on prostate cancer screening in black men. To address the barriers to prostate cancer screening for black men the Government has the power to:

- consider prostate cancer for black men as a public health priority;
- fund innovative and targeted campaign to encourage black men to go and get screened;
- ensure that mobile and intensive screening programmes exist to encourage participation for local people;
- ensure that prostate cancer guideline is produced to ensure that black men are referred by their doctors to get screened, regardless of perceived symptoms.
- follow up or come up with policies that are geared to address health inequalities. It will be advisable that the government work with these communities to understand better the kind of support they need to redress the imbalance in health inequalities;

- Provide resources to enable awareness and support initiatives to take roots and support the black community for the longer term;
- Work with black communities to ensure that all, regardless of the gender, play a role in tackling such inequalities.

Chapter 8
The Players

> *"It is a surprising and important gap, one that black men, women in our lives, health professionals, and policymakers can no longer afford to ignore."*

As black people, we have a very important role to play wherever we are. Individuals, families, communities, organisations and policymakers must play a central role in improving, protecting and sustaining the health of the population. By working each at our levels and at the same time together, we are able to effectively contribute to changing our behaviours as black people towards prostate cancer, increasing screening, thus lowering the morbidity and mortality associated with prostate cancer.

This obviously requires creating an enabling environment that facilitates behaviour change and removes the barriers that prevent black men from getting screened for prostate cancer. For instance, for intervention and engagement to be effective, all players – individuals, families, communities, organisations and policymakers – must understand the issue of prostate cancer in black men including the risk factors, the high mortality rate, the low survival rate and the barriers to screening.

Additionally, an aggressive and positive engagement to promote prostate cancer prevention among black men, as well as institutional screening policy, has the potential to increase early detection and reduce morbidity and mortality among this population group.

The Co-conspirators

> *"Cross the river in a crowd, and the crocodile won't eat you."*
>
> *- African proverb*

We Black Men, one to another and one to many, have the most essential role to play. As the Intervention and Engagement Model shows, we black men of all generations need to improve our knowledge of, change our negative attitudes, behaviours, and beliefs towards prostate cancer to give ourselves the chance to live longer.

The African man is seen as strong and macho. Generations of men are taught about strength and pride. This has to a great extent impacted on the ego, leading to men not addressing their feelings, talking about their health and wellbeing. When men get together, they talk about football, politics, girls and any other topics that are not personal. These attitudes need to change. We need to take the initiative to understand that we need to be our own co-conspirators.

The statistics about prostate cancer in black men are clear and staggering, 1 in 4 of us is likely to be diagnosed with prostate cancer. That is why it is important and beneficial for us to get screened and get treated sooner rather than waiting until it is in the late stages.

We need to listen to ourselves, to others' messages and efforts, to those who care about us. We need to take the role of the 'co-conspirator' to educate ourselves, to increase our confidence and tackle this issue and many others head-on.

This is, by no means, an easy journey to take. However, black men can learn to put their health first.

Someone says: *"the fear of the unknown cannot hurt us because we don't know it."* It is without a doubt that the decision to get screened for prostate cancer is a big one. It requires confidence and support, knowing that it could go either way. However, better be diagnosed earlier than later to give oneself the chance to prolong one's life.

There are many people in the black community who believe that using a role model from the black community, who can share a personal experience of prostate cancer, is highly significant in changing behaviour and improving black men screening rate.

The Protagonists

The women in our lives are the protagonists or the necks. They have the influence and can assume the central role in influencing black man's behaviour to take action. It is the biggest source of support and comfort.

> *"Where a woman rules, streams run uphill."*
> *~ Ethiopian proverb*

Wives or partners, sisters, mothers, grandmothers, daughters – whether they know it or not, have a significant role to play.

Women know very well that men, in general, are more reluctant to visit a doctor than women.

Considering the situation and the likelihood that families and friends might lose a close one because they are not screened much earlier for prostate cancer, every one of us has a responsibility to raise awareness about the issue and change the perceptions, behaviours, and attitudes of the black male population.

Women, most particularly partners, can use their influence to help encourage change in black men health-related behaviours and increase the number of black men who get screened for prostate cancer, particularly when it comes to talking about prostate cancer issues which black men consider intimate.

Women need to reassure their partners that the latter should not worry much and that he is not alone to face whatever health challenge thrown to him. Women can accompany their partners to the doctor and any other related appointment for support if needed. This can help their partners to loosen up and talk about their worries and fears.

We should not forget that for every black man who has prostate cancer there is a wife, a partner, a sister a daughter or granddaughter who suffers too. From the moment a black man is diagnosed with prostate cancer, this means life has changed for himself, his partner and his family. In some cases, life has changed forever. I can hear those stories in my head of women relating their experiences when their husbands or boyfriend was diagnosed with the disease. How life might have been from the first appointment to the doctor and to the treatment.

No women should have to tell such story one day because her partner was diagnosed with prostate cancer at a later stage and did not survive. Women can help avoid this. Let us not imagine the worse by ensuring we mobilise the community, getting fully involved in raising awareness and increase the uptake in screening.

Here are some practical ways in which women can help the men in their lives:

1. You can't expect someone to go out of their way to listen to what you have to say if you are shouting. You're shouting at them. It might be an emergency, but bad language is a definite no-no.

2. Pick a time that's convenient for both of you
Even my children don't wake me at 3 a.m. to share their anxieties or a painful rejection. They'd be welcome, but they respect my needs and know that they're more likely to command my full attention (and therefore

get the best nurturing and advice I have to offer) if they wait until after breakfast. If you don't expect – or worse, demand – selfless giving from your spouse, you're more likely to get what you really need.

3. Open with the positive

A patient told me recently about a failed attempt she'd made to improve communication between her and her husband. She began the conversation by saying, "You have a history of not listening to me, so I've adopted some strategies in the hope of getting through to you." Needless to say, her overture was poorly received.

4. Do not tell – use questioning and suggestion techniques a couple of examples would be:

"I would like to get your point of view on having a health MOT. I need your help with what just happened. Do you have a few minutes to talk?"

"Can we talk about medical check-ups? I think we have different perceptions about it. I would like to hear your thinking on this."

Additionally, women can use women's forums or support groups to spread the message to other women to ensure as many black men as possible get screened for prostate cancer before it is too late. Below I share a story of one woman who has written a book about dealing with her husband's diagnosis.

"Prostate cancer is not an automatic death sentence, and it certainly is not the death of intimacy in a relationship. My husband's diagnosis gave us an opportunity to grow and learn together. Even more than that, it provided an incentive to live life to the fullest and never let pass any opportunities to express love. Glenda's book, What Men Won't Talk About and Women Need to Know, chronicles her husband's prostate cancer journey from a woman's perspective."
-Gelnda Standeven

Her book is listed in my further reading chapter if you would like to read more and get some ideas.

The Confederate

Community Members - the community is important for many of us. It is an important source of confidence, understanding, strength, friendship and social norms that might help to influence behaviour. The community approaches and awareness to increase the prostate cancer screening is likely to take into consideration cultural and religious sensitivities and needs. Communities' message can be powerful and have a big effect on the individual. Communities have the opportunity to discuss the issue of prostate cancer openly in their events or gatherings.

Members of the community, prostate cancer survivors, owing to their experiences, have an even bigger role to play. They have a better understanding of the symptoms, what to do, where to go, and what other supports are available or helpful.

Black men love food and enjoy a good chat about football and politics. An innovative approach would be to replace those conversations with health and wellbeing discussions with the aim of breaking down barriers to communication. If you are a co-conspirator in your camp, start the subject. Do not wait for someone else to take the lead. I have tried this, and often the subject has been well received if more of us were co-conspirators and role models.

As the world is changing, there are more opportunities for men and women to sit in the same room and have conversations. This development opens up another great chance to talk about prostate cancer. Events with both men and women included individuals of both genders.

Increase outreach, targeting the black men and their families and communities. Invite black men to be involved in advertisements.

The Ecclesiastic Anchors

Religious and Community Leaders – religious and community leaders' roles are important. People are likely to listen to their congregation and community leaders. They have many resources at their disposal, different from other players. For instance, religious leaders can convey positive and reassuring messages to the community or congregation. Many religions promote good health and wellbeing. For instance, there is evidence in the Bible, the Quran, and other sacred texts that advise on the importance of maintaining good health as commanded by God and practiced by prophets and messengers.

The religious leaders, in particular, can use these religious texts that reinforce positive health behaviours. Religious leaders should:

- Promote responsible behaviour that respects the dignity of all persons and defends the sanctity of life;
- Increase public knowledge and influence opinion;

- Redirect charitable resources for spiritual and social care;
- Encourage and initiate discussions and action from the grassroots up to the national level.

There is also an opportunity to increase dialogue by including health awareness days in men's groups. These are usually multi-ethnic conversations which are great in opening up the dialogue at a wider level.

Chapter 9
What Next?

The reality of prostate cancer in black men is that they have poorer outcomes than white men and that 1 in 4 black men is likely to have prostate cancer in their lifetime.

There are many kinds of intervention that can be provided to help black men to engage and make the relevant and informed decisions. We can raise awareness of prostate cancer and influence black men's attitudes, behaviours and perspectives towards prostate cancer. The Intervention and Engagement Model mentioned in chapter 8, highlights different levels of interventions and the roles played by the actors involved.

Undoubtedly, there is a need to conduct awareness-raising campaigns to educate black communities, most particularly black men about the risk of getting prostate cancer. At policy level, a resolute approach is needed to encourage early screening amongst black men as well as improve and challenge the barriers across the prostate cancer care pathway.

For any intervention to be successful, many actors are needed to play an active role. This includes women, mainly partners. As a partner, women have the power of influence. She can be a source of support and comfort, the carer, the companion, and so on.

To achieve anything in life, engagement must be the top priority. I am ending this book by giving everyone some ideas of how black men can be better engaged. To improve their health outcomes:

1. Build a list of black role models. Use that to keep open channels of communication and send out regular surveys to get honest feedback about the issues black men face. It is called real listening.
2. Always act on the feedback and survey results - Let's say you survey your employees monthly

to find out how they're feeling. While some of their desires and wishes might be difficult to act on, send them updates explaining the progress you've made towards addressing their concerns even if it's just sending out a letter or email once in three months.

3. Build more trust - Overbearing doctors, wives, friends who are constantly 'nagging' might just be the fastest way to create disengagement and defensiveness. Trust them to realise the importance of looking after their health without checking if they have been to the clinic every day or dragging them kicking and screaming.

4. Consider Maslow's Hierarchy of Needs, once I was told to start a group to teach people about HIV prevention, without really considering what the people's basic needs were and looking at ways that would be improved. The result was catastrophic. Treat black men as people with all other needs too. Demonstrate genuine care by finding out what is going on in their lives.

5. Encourage health talks. Give black men more responsibility for their own health, not just more things you want them to do, in addition to their busy schedule.

6. Give them ownership of event planning events. Who has a better handle on the events black men will love than the black men themselves? Instead of trying to think of what you should do for them, involve them in the planning process, collaborate in finding the solution to engagement woes.

7. Clarify the purpose of your intervention. Give them 'inside' information. It is like any other part of life if you want to get your team more involved and committed to an intervention? Keep them informed. These are things like the direction of treatments, new research results, and any challenges.

8. Praise the co-conspirators – Protagonists know when your men have taken even the smallest step to seek help and get checked. Praise them, encourage them and appreciate when you hear about your partner's effort to make a life-changing decision like checking your health. Personally, congratulate them. It'll mean a lot to them and boost that man 'ego'. They are likely to do more which might lead to greater breakthroughs.

9. Do something fun, have more fun in life, "*life is too short right?*" Develop mentorship

programmes to coach, inspire and other men, especially the younger population. Encouraging black men to commit to community and social engagement by giving them the opportunity to participate in community service.

10. Invite a motivational speaker with a purpose to your next event, make it educational. Shake up the party, start it with inspiration. Everyone will be appreciative of the opportunity to grow and learn from whizzes. Maybe start a meeting with a brainstorm.

11. Offer healthier options such as health MOTs, health days, health retreats. This creates a great opportunity to pick up any other health issues that one may be experiencing. Promote perks that increase psychological and physical wellbeing and increase happiness. A happy person is more likely to take good care of themselves than an unhappy one.

12. Send out some Monday Motivation - Find an inspirational quote or page from a book and send it out to your team on Monday mornings. It's a super easy way to get people motivated and inspired and a day that's typically slow to start.

13. Transparency of communication and the integrity of the professionals' commitment to their health and for the black man not just being seen as just another unfortunate group. See them as partners, collaborators and not people to feel sorry for. Human interaction, social activities that engage our people as human beings in the human side of being part of a vibrant, growing, thriving culture.

14. Know something about the cultures and take time to learn one or two things about the person's lifestyle. It might give you a better handle on how you can be of help.

15. Let them make informed decisions and accept their wishes, in some cases no amount of education or intervention will get a black man to the door of the clinics if they are not in a critical condition. Nonetheless, if all the co-conspirators, protagonists, communities, religious leaders, and professionals have done their part, it fair to say the ball is in the black man's court.

Acknowledgements

This book is the result of a number of discussions I had with many black men and women around the issues of prostate cancer in black men. The journey started when I was researching for my master's degree in Public Health. Because of the idea of writing this book, which came from my lovely and amazing wife, I went out and talked to more black people – as individuals and in groups – and gather their thoughts, understanding, and experience of prostate cancer.

As a believer, I would like to express my gratitude to God almighty for his love, guidance, and mercy upon me, for my wonderful family and those who have helped me throughout my life.

I would wholeheartedly like to thank my wife without whose utmost and invaluable encouragement, advice, and support throughout this journey, this work would not have seen the light. I would also like to appreciate her for putting up with me and pushing me during those moments when I felt discouraged, and for being a source of inspiration and comfort.

I would like to thank my daughters, Naila Abdoul and Iman Abdoul for being amazing, cute, fun and a source of motivation, strength, and comfort.

Finally, I would also like to acknowledge every one of the many and extraordinary black men and women I talked to for their time and contribution, one way or another, to this book, and for helping make the journey excitingly stimulating.

Further Readings

If you would like to dig deeper and learn more about prostate cancer or black men in general, there are some books on Amazon that you can read. Here are a few:

1. Pushing through Fear Stereotypes and Imperfections: How to COACH Yourself Through Life's CHALLENGES and Boost Your MENTAL HEALTH by Amina Chitembo

2. What Men Won't Talk About . . . And Women Need to Know: A Woman's Perspective on Prostate Cancer Paperback – 31 Jul 2014 by Glenda Standeven.

3. Prostate Cancer - Stories of Men and Women: "My positive attitude helped!" Paperback – 15

Jul 2015 by Dr. Laurence Lepherd (Author), Dr. Coralie Graham (Editor)

4. The 2018-2023 World Outlook for Prostate Cancer Treatments and Prevention Paperback – 18 Dec 2017 by Icon Group International

5. The Black Man's Guide Out of Poverty: For Black Men Who Demand Better Paperback – 9 Feb 2015 by Aaron Clarey

References

Acheson, D. (1998). *Independent inquiry into inequalities in health*. London, The Stationery Office.

Agalliu et al. (2015). *The feasibility of epidemiological research on prostate cancer in African men in Ibadan, Nigeria*. BMC Public Health. (April). 15(425). Available at http://bmcpublichealth.biomedcentral.com/articles/10.1186/s12889-015-1754-x

American Cancer Society (2013). *Cancer Facts & Figures for African Americans 2013-2014*. Atlanta: American Cancer Society.

Arab L, Su J, Steck SE, et al. *Adherence to World Cancer Research Fund/American Institute for Cancer Research Lifestyle Recommendations Reduces Prostate Cancer Aggressiveness Among*

African and Caucasian Americans. Nutrition and Cancer. 65(5) 633-43.

Black, D., Morris,J.N., Smith.C. and Townsend, P. (1980). *Inequalities in Health: The Black Report.* London: Penguin

Bloom, J. R. et al. (2006). *Family History, Perceived Risk, and Prostate Cancer Screening among African American Men.* Cancer Epidemiology Biomarkers & Prevention: American Association for Cancer Research. (November).15(11). 2167- 2173. Available at http://cebp.aacrjournals.org/content/15/11/2167.full

Brawley, O.W. (2003). *Introduction: Cancer and health disparities. Cancer and Metastasis.* Kluwer Academic Publishers. 22(1). 7–9. Also available at https://link.springer.com/article/10.1023/A%3A1022299532270

Cancer Research UK (2014). *Prostate cancer survival statistics.* http://www.cancerresearchuk.org/health-professional/cancer-statistics/statistics-by-cancer-type/prostate-cancer/survival#YUrQW2gHz3f4ZAYq.99

Davey-Smith, G., Morris, J.N. and Shaw, M. (1998). The independent inquiry into inequalities in health. *British Medical Journal* 317: 1465-1466.

Department of Health (2011) *Improving Outcomes: A Strategy for Cancer*. DH. Also available at https://www.gov.uk/government/uploads/system/uploads/attachment_data/file/213785/dh_123394.pdf

Ford, M. E., Vernon, S. W., Havstad, S. L., Thomas, S. A., and Davis, S. D, (2006) Factors Influencing Behavioral Intention Regarding Prostate Cancer Screening among Older African-American Men. *Journal of the National Medical Association*. (98) 4: 505-514.

Garvan Institute (2013). CANCER – PROSTATE. http://www.garvan.org.au/research/diseases-we-research/cancer-prostate?gclid=CMjSr5vRh88CFRWeGwodXb0DpA

Haroon Siddique, H. (2015) *Prostate cancer twice as likely to kill black men as white men, study finds.* The Guardian. (July). Available at http://www.theguardian.com/society/2015/jul/30/prostate-cancer-twice-likely-kill-black-men-white-men-study

Hounsome, L. and Verne, J. (2012). *Mortality from Prostate Cancer*. South West Public Health Observatory

http://changingminds.org/explanations/belief/health_belief_model.htm

http://communityjournal.net/black-men-more-at-risk-for-prostate-cancer-have-this-in-common/

http://m.yorkshireeveningpost.co.uk/news/latest-news/top-stories/prostate-cancer-alert-as-leeds-named-as-worst-in-uk-for-early-diagnosis-in-black-men-1-7399763

http://mdquit.org/health-behavior-models/health-belief-model

http://recapp.etr.org/recapp/index.cfm?fuseaction=pages.TheoriesDetail&PageID=13

http://surroundhealth.net/Topics/Education-and-Learning-approaches/Behavior-change-strategies/Articles/Using-the-Health-Belief-Model-in-Different-Fields.aspx

http://time.com/3978319/prostate-cancer-black-men/

http://www.cancerresearchuk.org/health-professional/cancer-statistics/statistics-by-cancer-type/prostate-cancer/incidence

http://www.cancerresearchuk.org/health-professional/cancer-statistics/statistics-by-cancer-type/prostate-cancer#heading-Two

http://www.cbsnews.com/news/black-men-prostate-cancer-care/

http://www.cdc.gov/cancer/prostate/statistics/race.htm

http://www.dailymail.co.uk/health/article-
   3178699/Black-men-TWICE-likely-develop-
   prostate-cancer-white-men-study-warns
   .html

http://www.dailymail.co.uk/health/article-
   4655548/Prostate-cancer-deadly-black-men-
   gene.html

http://www.euromedinfo.eu/the-health-belief-
   model.html/

http://www.exeter.ac.uk/news/featurednews/
   title_437807_en.html

http://www.harvardprostateknowledge.org/
   prostate-cancer-risk-in-african-americans

http://www.med.upenn.edu/hbhe4/part2-ch3-
   main-constructs.shtml

http://www.medscape.com/viewarticle/726766

http://www.mirror.co.uk/news/uk-news/
   black-men-less-willing-tested-5256464

http://www.nhs.uk/be-clear-on-cancer/
   prostate-cancer

http://www.nhs.uk/Conditions/Cancer-of-the-
   prostate/Pages/Diagnosis.aspx

http://www.onlyanurse.com/nursingtopics/2015/
   1/19/the-health-belief-model-prostate-cancer-
   screening

http://www.uptodate.com/contents/active-surveil-
   lance-for-men-with-early-prostate-cancer

https://profiles.uonbi.ac.ke/gmagoha/publica-
    tions/overview-prostate-cancer-indigenous-
    black-africans-and-blacks-african-ancestr-0

https://www.cancer.org/cancer/prostate-cancer/
    detection-diagnosis-staging/how-diagnosed.
    html

Hubley, J. and Copeman, J. (2013). *Practical
    Health Promotion*. London: Polity Press

Hugh M. H. (1997). *Why Do African- American
    Men Suffer More Prostate Cancer?* Journal of
    the National Cancer Institute. (February).
    89(3). 188-189. Available at http://jnci.
    oxfordjournals.org/content/89/3/188.full.
    pdf+html

Katherine E. Smith, Clare Bambra, and Sarah E.
    Hill (2015). *Health Inequalities: Critical Per-
    spectives*. Oxford: Oxford University Press.

Kleier, J. A. 2003). *Prostate cancer in black men
    of African-Caribbean descent*. Journal of
    Cultural Diversity. PubMed. 10(2). 56-61.
    Available at http://search.proquest.com/
    docview/219312599/fulltextPDF/1261274C
    78694E63PQ/1?accountid=14693

Lina Jandorf, Matthew S. Chang, Kayode Smith,
    Alexis Florio, Simon J. Hall (2007). *Com-
    munity-Based Free Prostate Cancer Screening*

Program. Progress in Community Health Partnerships. 3:215-30.

Lloyd, T. et al (2015). *Lifetime risk of being diagnosed with, or dying from, prostate cancer by major ethnic group in England 2008–2010.* BMC Medicine. (July). 13(171). Available at http://bmcmedicine.biomedcentral.com/articles/10.1186/s12916-015-0405-5

Marmot, M., (2001). From Black to Acheson: two decades of concern with inequalities in health. A celebration of the 90th birthday of Professor Jerry Morris. *International Journal of Epidemiology*, 30(5), pp.1165-1171. Also available at: https://academic.oup.com/ije/article/30/5/1165/724201/From-Black-to-Acheson-two-decades-of-concern-with

Mofolo et al. (2015) *Knowledge of prostate cancer among males attending a urology clinic, a South African study.* Springer Plus. (February). 4(67). Available at http://www.springerplus.com/content/4/1/67

Nick Stockton, N. (2014). *Vitamin D may be key to why black men get more deadly prostate cancers.* Available at http://qz.com/204932/vitamin-d-may-be-key-to-why-black-men-get-more-deadly-prostate-cancers/

Obinna, C. (2015). *Why prostate cancer affects black men*. Available at http://www.vanguardngr.com/2015/09/why-prostate-cancer-affects-black-men-more

Obu, R. N. (2014). *Prostate Cancer: West African Men And The Trans-Atlantic Slave Trade, Any Connection With The High Incidence Rates?* https://www.modernghana.com/news/587729/prostate-cancer-west-african-men-an.html

Odedina, F. T. (2009). *Prostate cancer disparities in Black men of African descent: a comparative literature review of prostate cancer burden among Black men in the United States, Caribbean, United Kingdom, and West Africa*. BioMed Central. Available at http://www.ncbi.nlm.nih.gov/pmc/articles/PMC2638461/

Oliver, A. and Exworthy, M. (2003). *HEALTH INEQUALITIES Evidence, policy and implementation Proceedings from a meeting of the Health Equity Network*. London: The Nuffield Trust.

Oliver, J. S. (2008). *"Prostate Cancer Screening Patterns among African American Men in the Rural South"*. Dissertation, Georgia State University. http://scholarworks.gsu.edu/nursing_diss/7

OpenStax (2012). *Theoretical Perspectives on Social Stratification.* OpenStax CNX. http://cnx. org/contents/65d28eb1-2115-4291-9e00-67b76e61e121@2 .

Orji, R. Vassileva, J. Mandryk, R. (2012). *Towards an Effective Health Interventions Design: An Extension of the Health Belief Model.* Online Journal of Public Health Informatics. 4(3):e9. http://ojphi.org

Pinthus J.H., Pacik D., Ramon J. (2007) *Diagnosis of Prostate Cancer.* In: Ramon J., Denis L.J. (eds) Prostate Cancer. Recent Results in Cancer Research, vol 175. Springer, Berlin, Heidelberg. Also available at https://link.springer.com/chapter/10.1007/978-3-540-40901-4_6

Rajbabu, K. et al. (2007). *Racial origin is associated with poor awareness of prostate cancer in UK men, but can be increased by simple information.* Nature Publishing Group. 10, 256–260. Available at http://www.nature.com/pcan/journal/v10/n3/full/4500961a.html

Rebbeck, T. R. et al. (2013). *Patterns of Prostate Cancer Incidence, Aggressiveness, and Mortality in Men of African Descent.* Hindawi Publishing Corporation. Volume 2013. Available at http://www.hindawi.com/journals/pc/2013/560857/

Reynolds, D. (2008) *Prostate Cancer Screening in African American Men: Barriers and Methods for Improvement.* American Journal of Men's Health. SAGE. 2(2). 172-177. Also available at http://jmh.sagepub.com/content/2/2/172

Scutti, S. (2015). *Black Men In The UK Have Double The Risk Of Prostate Cancer, Compared To White Men.* Available at http://www.medicaldaily.com/black-men-uk-have-double-risk-prostate-cancer-compared-white-men-345224

World Cancer Research Fund International/ American Institute for Cancer Research Continuous Update Project Report (2014). *Diet, Nutrition, Physical Activity, and Prostate Cancer.* Available at: http://www.wcrf.org/sites/default/files/Prostate-Cancer-2014-Report.pdf

Final Remarks

Firstly, thank you for taking time to read my book. Your reviews are important to me. So here is my request. If you enjoyed this book and learned something from it, you can help me in one or more of the following ways:

→ Go online, at www.amazon.co.uk or my website www.aliabdoul.com, write a kind review.

→ Let us connect on Social Media:

  ○ **LinkedIn:** https://www.linkedin.com/in/ali-abdoul

  ○ **Facebook:** https://www.facebook.com/ali.aw.abdoul

→ Attend one of my trainings or seminars

→ Email me if I can be of any help with your training or awareness raising events ali@diverse-cultures.co.uk. I do reply directly.

→ Get a copy of this book as a gift to your friend or family.

→ Continue to grow to the next level of your life and build the happy life and success you want.

THANK YOU FOR .

About the Author

Ali Abdoul is a UK based **Public Health Community Inclusion Specialist, Author**, **Trainer**, and **Speaker** who specialises in Black Men's Health, Community Inclusion, Equality and Diversity.

He has more than 20 years' experience helping policy makers, mainstream leaders, and communities to collaborate and promote community cohesion, health and well-being through inclusion, advocacy, and educational programmes, using multidisciplinary approaches.

He is married and has two daughters and two older step daughters and enjoys reading and researching.

Training/Speaking/Seminar Topics: (1) Public Health Inclusion: Black Men's Health, (2) Equality and Diversity, (3) Community Development.

Books written or co-authored including current book:
Celebrating Diversity: Positive Stories of Migration from Around the World.

Company/Business Name: Diverse Cultures Ltd

Contact Details:
LinkedIn: https://www.linkedin.com/in/ali-abdoul
Facebook: https://www.facebook.com/ali.aw.abdoul
Phone: +44 (0) 7397010685
Email: Ali@diverse-cultures.co.uk | aawa.abdoul@gmail.com
Websites: www.aliabdoul.com | www.diverse-cultures.co.uk

SUBSCRIBE TO MY BLOG:
Get more training, tools and tips from me and other thought leaders on Inclusion issues:
https://www.aliabdoul.com
I will see you there.
—Ali.

Made in the USA
Coppell, TX
14 June 2021